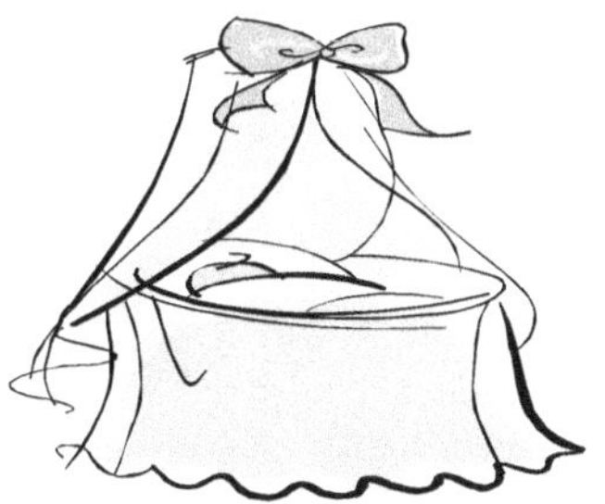

Place of Birth (Hospital):

____

City:________________________State:____________

Phone: (______)____________________________

Doctor / Nurse Name:

____

Mother's Name & Phone Number:

____

(______)________________________________

Father's Name & Phone #:

____

(______)________________________________

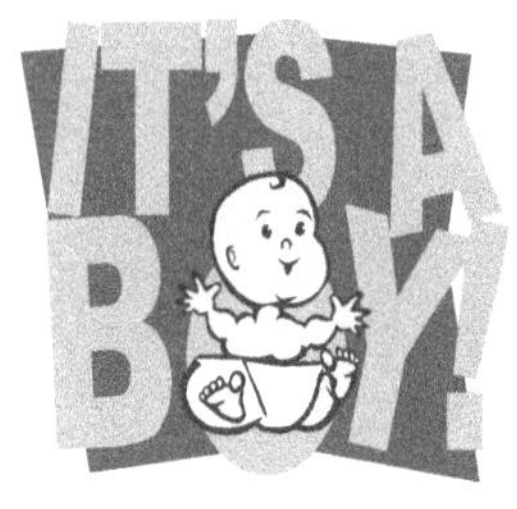

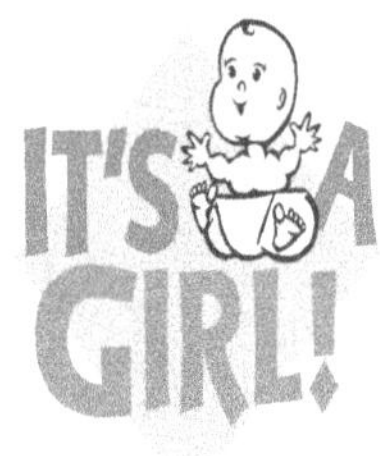

Welcoming Baby:
(BOY / GIRL)

____

Date of Birth:

____

Time of Birth:

____ (A.M. / P.M.)

Weigh:

________ Lbs.. ________ oz. ________ inches

Number of Weeks Gestation:

____

Number of Days Spent in Hospital:

____

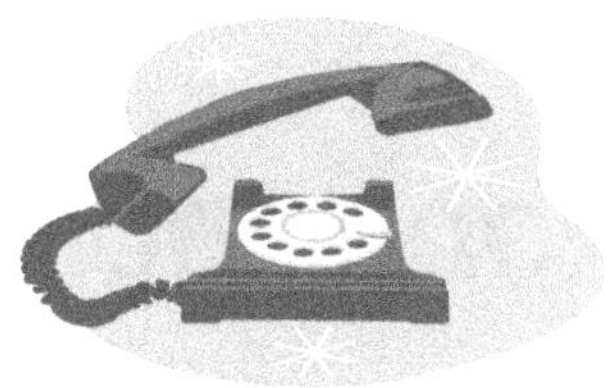

Emergency Contact - Name & Phone #:

____

(   ) ______________________________________

Doctor - Name & Phone #:

____

(   ) ______________________________________

Pharmacy - Name & Phone #:

____

(   ) ______________________________________

Insurance - Name & Phone #:

____

(   ) ______________________________________

____

INTRODUCTION

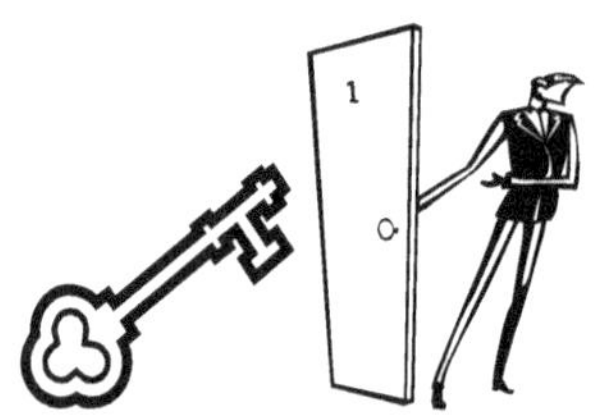

This book is dedicated to new parents that want vital, on the spot information about caring for their new premature infant.

Also for those that don't have time to read huge books, but need help right away on where to start.

I hope that my 24 week gestation, 1 pound, 11 oz. experience will help others in similar situations.

Once you have information to lead your preemie to grow strong and healthy everything else should fall in place.

Just remember to STAY STRONG! Your little miracle needs your love and support.

WELCOMING

Congratulations!

Congratulations! You have just delivered a little miracle baby. What a beautiful moment, also a scary feeling. You are now facing the reality of your new premature infant.

Too much to take in all at once? Each day will get better. I hope that my personal experiences can help you to cope through this stressful moment.

Do you feel alone because no one else knows what you have just been through emotionally?

Just remember to try your best to stay strong. Not just for you, but for your family. Save your strength to get through this very tense moment and to stay on top of things.

Don't even think about sitting back yet! There's a lot that you have to do. Giving birth to a preterm infant is a challenging and rewarding experience. You have been faced with a reality check that you didn't have time to prepare for.

Welcome to the real world –
YOUR NEW PREMATURE INFANT & YOU!

I remembered the fear of losing my infant during the first few days. Weeks later I experienced the excitement of preparing to bring him home. A place where just my family and me.

Depending on the gestational age and the overall medical condition, a premature infant may have to be transferred to the hospital's Neonatal Intensive Care Unit (NICU) sometimes called the Newborn Intensive Care Unit department.

Placing preemie infants in the hospital's NICU department is to provide them with specialized medical staff and equipment that is needed for the infant's specific medical needs.

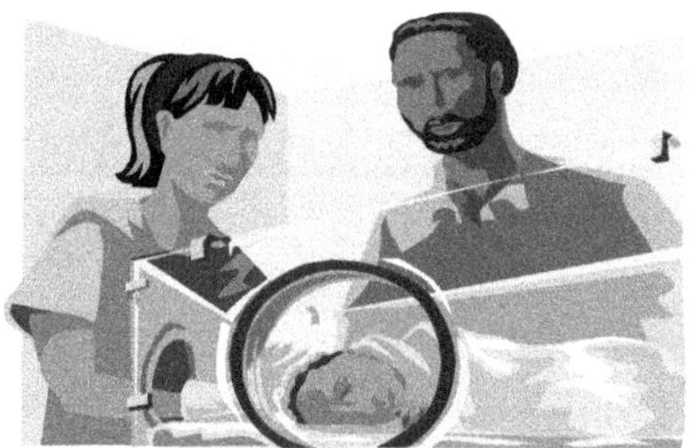

Low baby fat in preemie infants may cause their bodies to become colder in normal room temperature than full term infants, therefore your preemie may be placed in an incubator instead of a regular baby crib after birth to keep him/her warm or for other medical reasons.

Incubators are special beds for preemie infants that maintain a stable temperature by the use of a thermostat. Most preemie infants may be placed on a cardio respiratory monitor for breathing and heart rate.

Because of their lungs not being fully developed, extra oxygen and other special medical equipment may also be needed to help with breathing.

Talk to your doctor about keeping you informed about your preemie's health condition and of any changes that may occur.

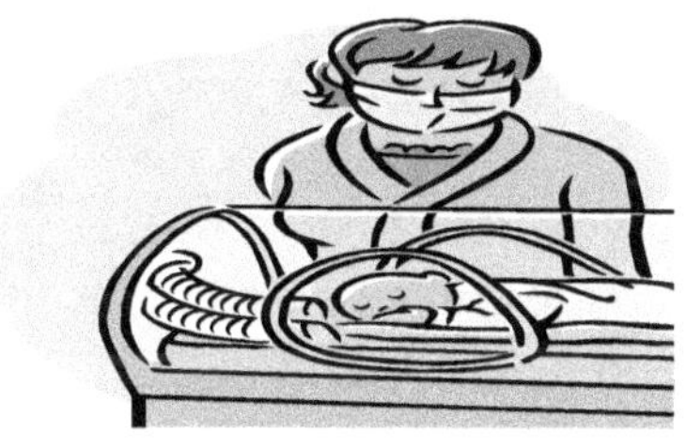

Get to know the nurses and other medical staff who are caring for your preemie. Don't be afraid to ask questions.

Appreciate the hospital staff for the work they provide to help care for your infant and you. They are very special people who are highly trained.

You have to trust them to do the right thing. Think about where you might be if you didn't have them around.

DON'T WAIT – DO IT NOW!

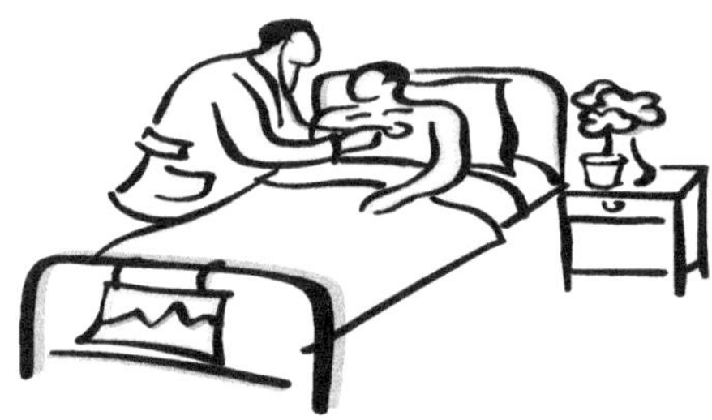

You're still at the hospital wondering what just happened? What are you going to do next? How are you going to do it?

You have things that you have to do now that your preemie is here. It's ok if you are still admitted in the hospital. This work requires your brain. Fast thinking!

Ask the hospital staff if it's ok to make local calls from your hospital bed.

Once you have the approval to do so you can start working on getting things done for your preemie with the help of this book.

CHOOSING A NAME:

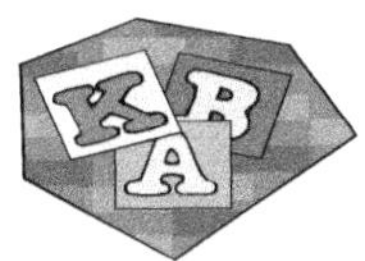

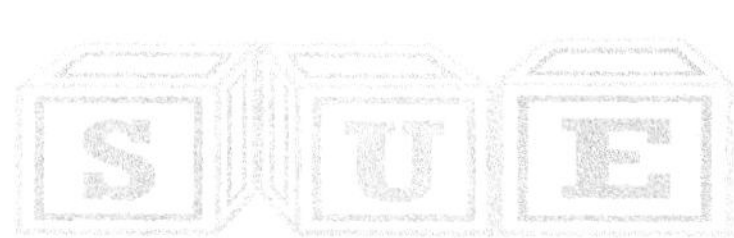

If you haven't already, choose a name for your new infant. A name and spelling that you and your family agree with.

Write it down and spread the word of your new infant's name with others.

1st Choice: ______________________________

____

2nd Choice: ______________________________

____

3rd Choice: ______________________________

____

Note: ______________________________

____

CONTACT YOUR HEALTH INSURANCE COMPANY

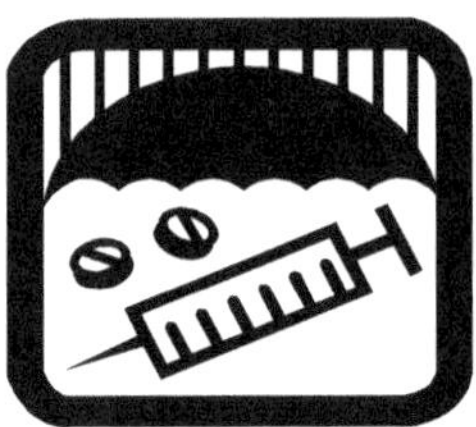

Add your new infant to your current insurance policy or set up a new policy. Inform your health insurance company of the preterm birth of your new infant.

Give the name, date and additional information needed in order to set your infant up for health insurance.

If your child was born under 2 lbs., your preemie might be eligible for Medicaid, regardless of your income.

Check in the reference chapter of this book for additional information about Medicaid benefits.

Notes: ____

____

____

____

SOCIAL SECURITY CARD

Check with the hospital staff first to see if they provide information about filing for a social security card for your new infant.

If not, call the Social Security Office at **800.773.1213** to set up information to receive a social security card for your infant.

You may also visit your local Social Security office or go online at www.ssa.gov to download application (**Form SS-5**).

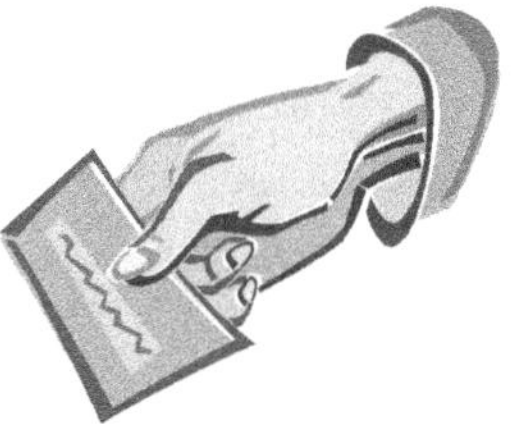

Get extra certified copies of your child's birth certification and hospital's birth records may be needed. GET IT NOW TO SAVE TIME LATER!

When you receive your infant's social security card store in a safe place. Be careful about sharing the social security number with others.

After your application is received at the administration office your infant's card should be mailed to you within a few weeks.

BIRTH CERTIFICATE:

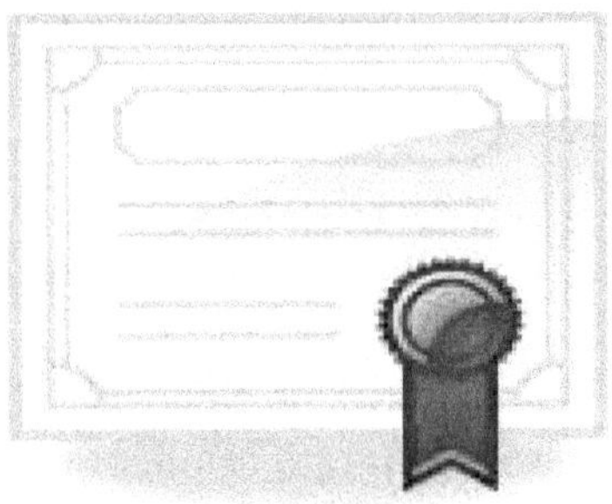

Ordering a Certified Copy of your new infant's Birth Certificate may be needed for health insurance, bank accounts, applying for a social security card and for other important reasons.

Ask the hospital if they have an onsite case worker for help on filing vital records for your new infant.

If the hospital doesn't offer this service then check with your local city / county vital records department about filing and receiving a certified copy of your infant's birth certificate.

Don't sit back yet. This is just the beginning of a busy project. It's best to know ahead of time instead of waiting until the last minute. Preparing early can save you from a lot of stress and confusion in the future.

QUESTIONS TO ASK YOUR DOCTOR BEFORE LEAVING THE HOSPITAL

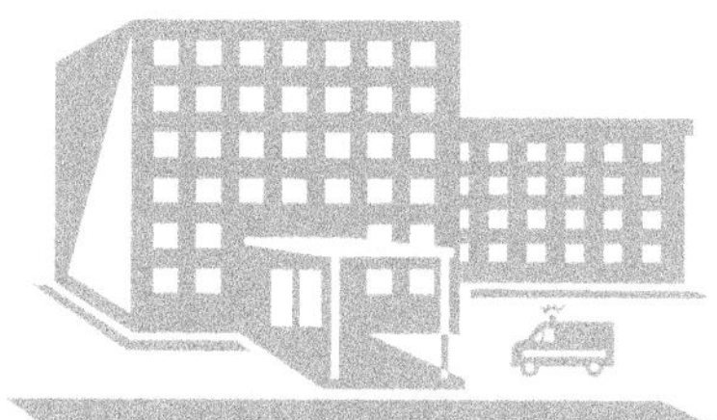

Leaving the hospital without your baby can make you feel empty. Remember that your infant is in a safe place and is being treated by a team of experienced and professionals.

You may have checked out of the hospital without your preemie, but this doesn't mean that you can't contact the hospital for current information about your infant's health status.

Information about your infant should be available to you (the parent) by phone 24 hours a day. Check the hospital where your preemie was born to verify the hospital's policy (privacy, rules, etc.) for visitations, etc.

ASK YOUR PREEMIE's MEDICAL STAFF:

- ✓ **Current conditions and health status.**
- ✓ **Estimated date for preemie to be discharged from the hospital.**
- ✓ **Medical equipment that may be needed when released from the hospital.**
- ✓ **Suggestions on training classes. Things to know and learn before preemie is discharged.**
- ✓ **Visiting time at the hospital for parents, family and friends.**
- ✓ **How many people will be allowed per visit.**
- ✓ **Description of special infant car seat that may be needed when discharged from the hospital.**

You have a ton of things to do before your preemie arrives home from the hospital. Prepare ahead of time to bring your preemie home to a safe, clean and loving environment.

SINCE YOUR LITTLE ONE ARRIVED EARLY:

- ____ **Set up your infant's crib / sleeping area.**

- ___ **Search for primary pediatrician and specialists. Research the doctor's background. Know and understand the practice of the specialist, etc.**

- ___ **Start early scheduling your appointments. Schedule appointments ahead of time before your preemie comes home. Some appointments could take weeks or even months just to see a doctor of your choice especially for new patients. You might be able to be seen sooner than your scheduled date if you call in to check for any cancellations.**

- ___ **Shop for preemie clothing, diapers, etc.**

- ___ **Shop for special bottles, formula, etc.**

- ___ **Training on medical equipment.**

- ___ **Proper training on feeding and caring for your preemie.**

- ___ **Medications needed. Understand medication usage and dosage, etc.**

- ____ **Prepare a list of important names, addresses and phone numbers of doctors, family members, etc.**

- ___ **Detailed cleaning of your preemie's bedroom. You want your house to be germ-free as possible to prevent your preemie from sickness.**

- ___ **Rest! Do it now while you can.**

Have you checked all? Good for You!

FACING REALITY

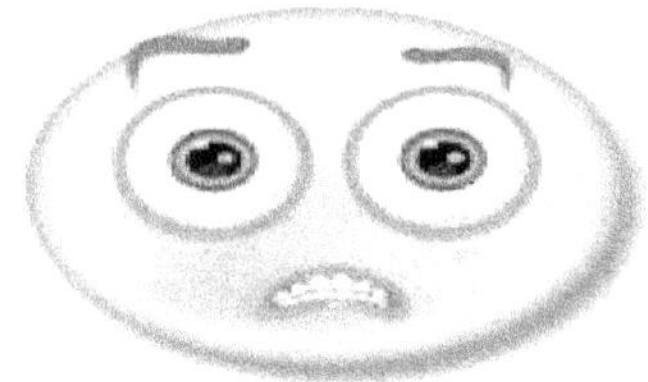

Learn how to ask for help from people you know and trust. You will need it. Get the help you need in order to care for your preemie.

Take time for yourself to THINK CLEARLY. That's correct, you need time to THINK! Take time to regroup.

All that you have been through, you need to clear your mind. Try to go on a vacation, finish old projects or something personal for yourself at home. Do it NOW while you can.

Treat yourself! You deserve it, plus you might not have much time for pampering when your preemie comes home. Having a baby is a lot of work, having a preemie is even more.

You can't really prepare yourself for all that's about to happen, just be ready for when it comes. Your preemie is depending on YOU!

Prepare yourself for this stronger, wiser and challenging new person that you are about to become. You will look back and appreciate every minute of it.

HOMEWORK ASSIGNMENT

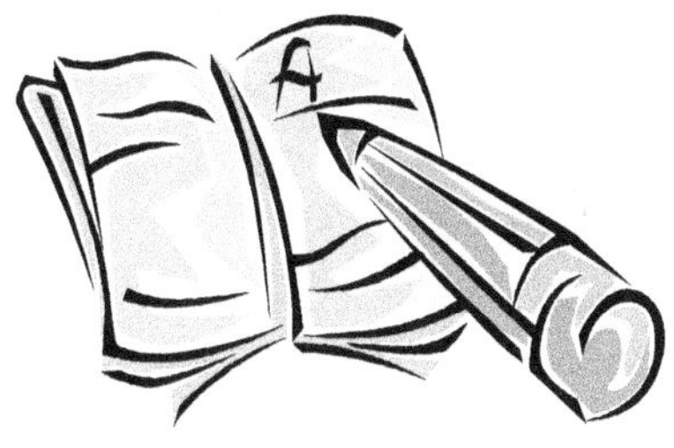

It's getting closer to the time for your preemie to come home. You have work that you have to do before your child arrives home. Be ready to take notes.

RESEARCH information about your child's medical condition. Go online, visit the library, read books, join support groups, organizations and other programs. Educate yourself as much as possible to learn more about your preemie.

Listen to what doctors and other medical professionals have to say about your child's health condition. Ask questions.

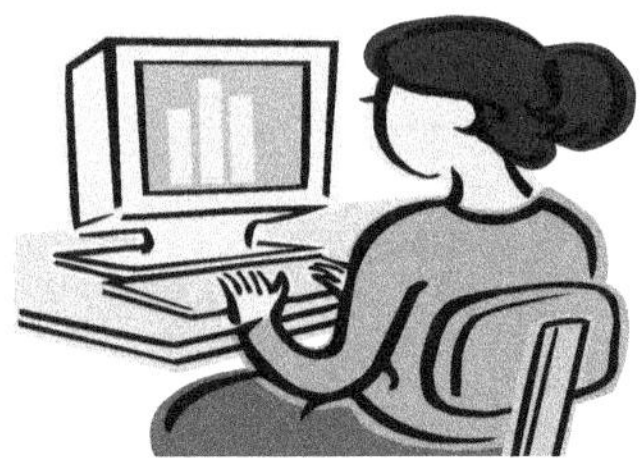

Take notes. If you don't understand ask additional questions and research information for yourself.

Talk to other parents in similar situations.

Learn how to use of your infant's car seat.

Learn how to use all of your preemie's medical equipment.

Understand medications given. Contact your infant's doctor if any changes occur during the use of any medication.

Program doctors, pharmacist, etc. in your cell phone.
Have a list of emergency contacts with you at all times.

Make yourself available. Keep an open schedule for your child in case of an emergency.

Remember you the parent might be the first to contact if your infant becomes sick while left with a babysitter, etc.

Keep hardcopy notes for backup in case you phone is lost.

PREEMIE'S DISCHARGED DAY FROM THE HOSPITAL

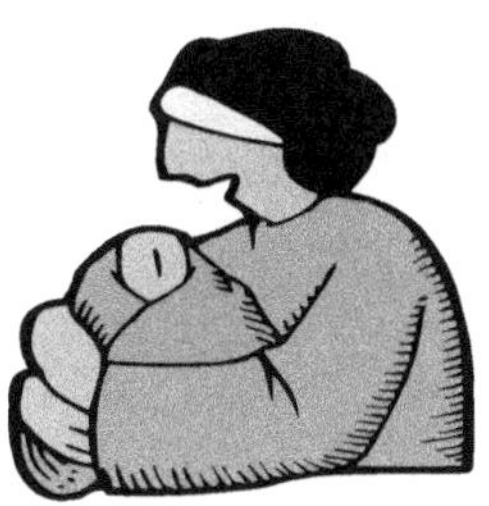

What a joy! You are feeling like a new mom again while carrying your preemie infant from the hospital to the car. Congratulations to you and your family.

This may be your preemie's first time outdoors in the weather. Make sure that your infant is dressed appropriately before leaving the hospital to protect him/her from the different climate. This is a big change for your preemie.

Bring appropriate clothing and blankets for changing your preemie before leaving the hospital.

Check with the medical staff at the hospital for suggestions.

ARRIVING HOME

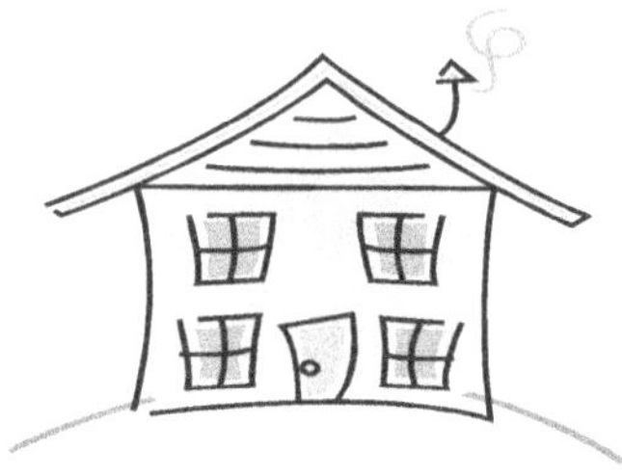

You are finally at home with your preemie infant. What a beautiful feeling to have you and your family together at home.

If you are not able to be there for your child 24 hours a day, someone else has to fill in to help. You will need to take a break sometimes.

Make arrangement for additional help. You will need it sooner or later. Either family, daycare centers or a private nurse. Interview now!

Make sure that you know and trust the person well enough to care for your preemie.

Be sure that they are fully aware and have proper training to care for your infant.

Try to handle all of your vital business and personal activities before time.

Here are some suggestions:

(Ask infant's doctor for recommendations)

- ❑ Limit Your Visitors. Try not to have too many new people around visiting your new infant until your preemie's immune system is strong enough.

- ❑ Avoid smoke. Please don't smoke around your new infant. Be sure to keep your clothing and room smoke-free around your preemie.

- ❑ Avoid Pets. Fleas, pet hair, etc. can be unsafe around your preemie. Wait until your child is stronger.

- ❑ Wash your hands. Get in the habit of washing your hands before and after handling your preemie.

- ❑ Help your preemie adjust to the new environment. Remember that your infant is no longer in the hospital.

- ❑ Keep on a dim light and a low volume radio.

- ❑ Schedule your preemie's feeding time. Talk to your infant's doctor about feeding instructions, diets, type of formulas, vitamins, etc. that's best for your preemie.

- ❑ Know your preemie's pharmacist and understand the use of medications.

- ❑ Keep a chart record of your infant's activities. Growth, first timers (crawl, steps, sit up), sleeping habits, health appointments, immunizations (shots), etc.

INSURANCE

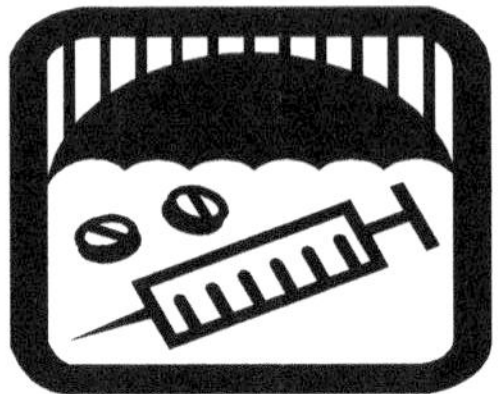

Know your copay for doctor's office visits and for prescription drugs. Information may be imprinted on your insurance card or you can go to your insurance's company's website (if available) to check for information online.

Regardless if you go online or call your insurance company directly, it is very important for you to know information about doctors, specialists, prescription drugs, hospital emergency visits, etc. that is covered under your plan.

It's best to first write down the name and additional information about your potential health professionals. Check with your insurance company to verify coverage plus your overall out of pocket expenses.

Just because you have health insurance doesn't mean that you are automatically covered for vision, dental or prescription drugs.

Take the time to check with your insurance company about what's included in your plan. You will be happy that you did.

Also remember that just because you may have prescription drugs coverage, this doesn't mean that all treatments will apply under your plan.

NOW YOUR PREEMIE's NEEDS

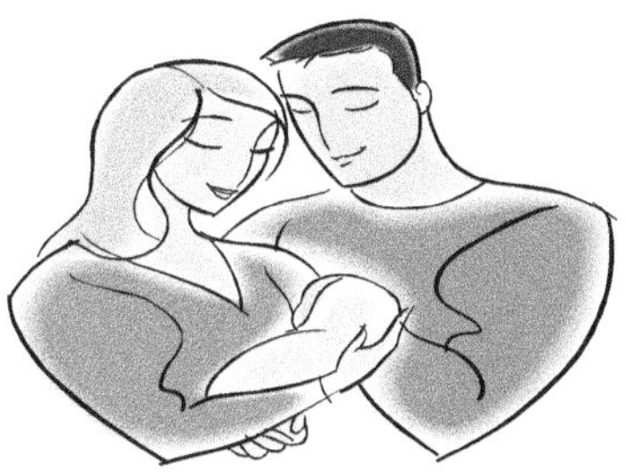

Enjoy every minute learning about your preemie. Knowing and learning about your infant's situation helps you to feel stronger and more secure.

Focus on your infant and not the disability. Study the strengths and weakness. Inform your infant's doctor of any concerns and changes.

Be around others for positive encouragement and don't be afraid to ask for help.

When your preemie comes home you may see him more than anyone else. Watch your baby closely. Ask your infant's doctor questions.

If you don't feel comfortable about the information given to you don't be afraid to get a second or even a third opinion. Remember no question is a stupid question. Just because some professionals hold specialized title, they may have different opinions that may not be best for your infant.

Educate yourself. Know your preemie's needs.

Information / Assistance

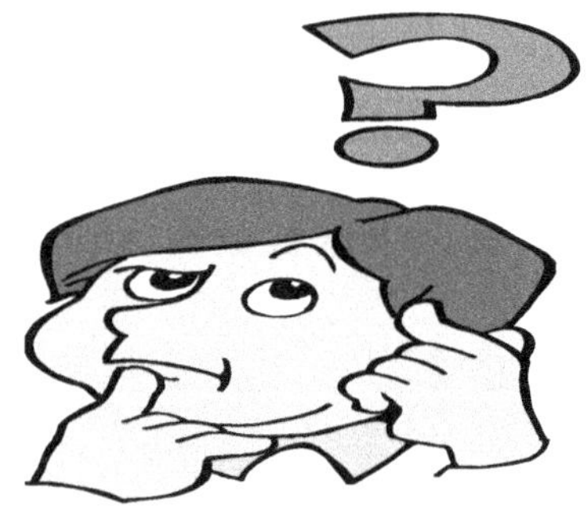

CARSEATS

Some hospitals / nonprofits give out free. Check your local area.

www.epao.org **www.healthlychildren.org**

EASTER SEALS

www.Easterseals.com

HEALTH INSURANCE

www.health.gov

Health Insurance Portability and Accountability Act (HIPPA)
www.hhs.gov/ocr/hippa

National Immunization Information

Phone: 800.232.4636 **www.cdc.gov**

MARCH OF DIMES

www.MarchofDimes.org

MEDICAID

In most cases, premature birth will be eligible for federal assistances.

www.Mediciaid.gov

MIRACLE BABIES

www.miraclebabies.org **Phone: 858-633-8540**

RONALD MCDONALD HOUSE

www.rmhc.org **Phone: 630-623-7048**

RSV PROTECTION

www.rsvprotection.com

SSI

Supplemental Security Income (SSI)

Phone: 800.772.1213 **www.ssi.gov**

Additional Notes:

www.ingramcontent.com/pod-product-compliance
Lightning Source LLC
LaVergne TN
LVHW010550100826
845148LV00013B/2679

* 9 7 8 0 9 7 7 3 9 2 0 4 9 *